MW01206558

COMPLETE GUIDE TO UNDERSTANDING HERNIA REPAIR

Comprehensive Insights, Procedures, Recovery Tips For Expert Techniques, Patient Care, And Post-Operative Healing Strategies

KLEIN HOYLE

© [KLEIN HOYLE] [2024]

All rights reserved.

Disclaimer

The content in this book is based on the author's expertise and comprehension of the topic. The author has no affiliation or link with any corporation, business, or person. This book is meant to give general information and educational material only, and it should not be interpreted as professional medical advice. Always seek the advice of a skilled healthcare expert if you have any queries about medical issues or treatments. The author and publisher expressly disclaim any responsibility resulting directly or indirectly from the use or use of the information included in this book.

Table of Contents

ABOUT THIS BOOK

The "Complete Guide to Understanding Hernia Repair" is an invaluable resource for patients, caregivers, and medical professionals alike, providing detailed insights into the complex world of hernias and their surgical treatment. In the first few chapters, readers are taken through the foundations of hernias, including their description, several varieties (such as inguinal, umbilical, and femoral), causes, and the telltale signs and symptoms that need care.

This book walks readers through the difficulties of hernia repair surgery, demystifying the procedure and arming them with information. From the contrasted procedures of open vs laparoscopic operations to the thorough preoperative examinations and preparations, every detail is carefully explained, offering a comprehensive comprehension for both patients and practitioners.

This book dissects each form of hernia with surgical precision, from the most common inguinal hernias to the rarer femoral hernias. By delving into the details of surgical treatments, readers learn about the anatomy, reasons, and unique dangers associated with each kind, allowing them to make educated choices about their care.

The emphasis on laparoscopic hernia repair procedures is particularly significant, since it heralds advances in less invasive surgery. Readers are taken to the cutting edge of current surgical innovation via extensive examinations of the benefits, procedures, and recovery results.

Furthermore, this book extensively covers the postoperative period, stressing the significance of individualized treatment and close monitoring. From immediate hospital care to long-term follow-up measures, every part of postoperative rehabilitation is painstakingly planned, assuring a smooth transition to recovery and normality.

Complications and hazards are unavoidable in the world of surgery, and this book tackles them front on. By shining light on possible dangers such as infection, recurrence, and persistent pain, it gives readers the foresight they need to face obstacles efficiently, instilling confidence and resilience.

In essence, the "Complete Guide to Understanding Hernia Repair" goes beyond the scope of a simple informative resource, emerging as a beacon of empowerment and enlightenment on the path to hernia treatment and recovery. It not only educates but also raises readers by bridging the gap between anxiety and certainty, bringing them along a road of educated decision-making and overall well-being.

CHAPTER 1

Introduction To Hernias

What Is A Hernia?

A hernia develops when an organ or tissue pushes through a weak area or ruptures in the surrounding muscle or connective tissue. Essentially, it looks like a bulge or ruptures in the abdominal wall or groin. This may happen for a variety of causes, including stress, muscular weakness, or injury.

Types Of Hernias Include Inguinal, Umbilical, And Femoral

There are several varieties of hernias, each called for its location and features. The most frequent varieties are inguinal hernias in the groin, umbilical hernias around the belly button, and femoral hernias in the upper thigh or groin.

Other forms include incisional hernias, which form at the site of a prior surgical incision, and hiatal hernias, which occur when the upper section of the stomach bulges through the diaphragm and into the chest cavity.

Inguinal hernias are the most common, accounting for about 70% of all hernias, and they occur more often in males than in women. Umbilical hernias are most often seen in newborns, although they may also develop in adults, particularly those who are overweight or pregnant. Femoral hernias are more frequent in women and are often caused by straining or carrying heavy things.

Causes And Risk Factors

A variety of conditions may contribute to the development of hernias. Weakness in the abdominal wall muscles is the major reason, which may be congenital (existing at birth) or acquired.

The following factors enhance the likelihood of getting a hernia:

• Heavy lifting, coughing, and straining during bowel movements might weaken abdominal muscles and lead to hernia development.

• Obesity strains the abdominal muscles, increasing the risk of weakness and herniation.

• Pregnancy may weaken abdominal muscles and cause hernias, especially umbilical hernias.

• Chronic coughing, such as from COPD or smoking, may strain abdominal muscles and raise the risk of hernias.

• Previous abdominal surgery: Incisions weaken the abdominal wall, increasing the risk of hernias if not properly healed and strengthened.

• The risk of hernias increases with aging as muscles weaken and tissues lose flexibility.

Symptoms Of Hernia

The symptoms of a hernia vary based on its nature and severity. Common symptoms include:

• A visible bulge or lump in the afflicted region, which may become more noticeable while standing, coughing, or straining.

• Experience pain or discomfort while carrying large things, coughing, or bending over.

• Heaviness or pressure in the abdomen or groin.

• The hernia may cause burning or painful sensations.

• Problems with bowel movement or urine, especially if the hernia is big or creating blockage.

• Nausea and vomiting may develop if the hernia causes intestinal blockage.

If you have persistent or severe hernia symptoms, you should seek medical assistance immediately, since untreated hernias may lead to consequences such as incarceration (the trapping of an intestinal loop in the hernia sac) or strangulation (the loss of blood flow to the trapped tissue).

CHAPTER 2

Understanding Hernia Repair Surgery

Overview Of Hernia Repair Surgery

Hernia repair surgery tries to repair a hernia, which arises when an organ pushes through a hole in the muscle or tissue that maintains it in position. The most frequent sort of hernia is in the abdomen, but they may also form in the groin, upper thigh, belly button, or even after surgical scars.

When a hernia develops, surgery may be required to relieve symptoms and avoid problems. The procedure consists of putting the bulging tissue back into position and mending the weakening muscle or tissue to avoid recurrence.

There are two main approaches to hernia repair surgery: open surgery and laparoscopic surgery. Each strategy has benefits and disadvantages, which we will discuss in the following sections.

Hernia Repair Techniques: Open Vs. Laparoscopic

Open hernia repair is a classic procedure in which the physician makes an incision directly over the hernia. The projecting tissue is pulled back into position, and any weakening muscles or tissues are strengthened with sutures or mesh. Open surgery gives the surgeon immediate access to the hernia, making it ideal for big or difficult hernias. However, it usually takes longer to heal and maybe more uncomfortable at first.

On the other side, laparoscopic hernia repair is a minimally invasive approach in which the surgeon creates small incisions and repairs the hernia using a tiny camera and specialized equipment. The camera offers a magnified picture of the region, enabling accurate repairs. When compared to open surgery, laparoscopic surgery often produces less discomfort, shorter hospital stays, and faster recovery. However, it may not be appropriate for all forms of hernias and might be technically difficult for certain surgeons.

Choosing between open and laparoscopic surgery is determined by many criteria, including the size and location of the hernia, the patient's general health, and the surgeon's experience. Your surgeon will go over the choices with you and propose the best technique for your unique condition.

Benefits And Risks Of Surgery

Hernia repair surgery has various advantages, including relief from pain, discomfort, and swelling, as well as a lower risk of complications linked with untreated hernias, such as intestinal obstruction or strangling. Surgical correction of the hernia attempts to restore normal function and avoid recurrence.

Hernia repair surgery, like any other surgical operation, is not without danger. Infection, hemorrhage, anesthetic response, nerve or blood vessel injury, and hernia recurrence are all possible complications. The chances of encountering these dangers vary based on the kind of operation, the surgeon's ability, and the patient's general condition.

To make an educated choice about whether surgery is suitable for you, you must first examine the possible risks and benefits with your healthcare professional.

Preparing For Hernia Repair Surgery

Preparing for hernia repair surgery entails various measures to guarantee a good result and a smooth recovery. Your surgeon will offer precise recommendations customized to your unique requirements; however, some broad suggestions may include:

1. Medical assessment: Before surgery, you will have a full medical assessment to examine your general health and detect any underlying disorders that may impair the operation or recovery process.

2. Preoperative Testing: Depending on your medical history and the kind of hernia, your surgeon may prescribe preoperative testing including blood tests, radiology scans, or electrocardiograms to assess your health and identify any possible issues.

3. Medication Management: Before surgery, your surgeon may advise you to discontinue certain medicines, such as blood thinners or nonsteroidal anti-inflammatory drugs (NSAIDs), to lower the risk of bleeding or other problems.

4. Fasting: To lessen the danger of aspiration during anesthesia, you will most likely be asked not to eat or drink for some time before to operation.

5. Lifestyle adjustments: Making lifestyle adjustments such as stopping smoking, keeping a healthy weight, and avoiding heavy lifting or stressful activities will help you maximize your health and get better surgery results.

6. Arrangements for Recovery: Plan ahead of time for your recovery by organizing transportation to and from the hospital, arranging for support at home during the first recovery period, and stocking up on necessities like pain pills and comfortable clothes.

By following your surgeon's instructions and properly preparing for surgery, you may help guarantee a good result and an easy recovery after hernia repair surgery.

CHAPTER 3

Preoperative Evaluation And Preparation

Medical History Assessment

Before having hernia repair surgery, it is critical to have a full medical history evaluation. This is a thorough conversation with your healthcare practitioner about your previous medical problems, surgeries, medicines, allergies, and any family history of hernias or other pertinent health concerns.

During this examination, your healthcare professional will ask questions to better understand your general health and any variables that may impact your operation or recovery. This includes questions concerning chronic conditions such as diabetes or hypertension, recent surgeries, and any drugs you are presently using, including over-the-counter vitamins.

The medical history evaluation also allows you to express any concerns or questions you have regarding the planned procedure. It is critical, to be honest and upfront throughout this talk to create the safest and most successful treatment plan customized to your specific requirements.

Physical Examination

A thorough physical examination is an important component in the preoperative assessment for hernia repair surgery. During this examination, your healthcare professional will visually evaluate and palpate the afflicted region to determine the hernia's size, location, and severity.

They will also assess your general health state, which includes vital indicators like blood pressure, heart rate, and temperature. They may also test your abdominal muscular strength and look for symptoms of problems like incarceration or strangulation.

The physical examination gives crucial information to your healthcare professional, allowing them to decide the best surgical strategy and method for hernia repair.

Diagnostic Tests Include Ultrasounds, Mris, And CT Scans

In addition to a medical history and physical examination, diagnostic testing such as ultrasound, MRI (Magnetic Resonance Imaging), or CT (Computed Tomography) scans may be requested to further analyze the hernia.

Ultrasound is a non-invasive imaging technology that uses high-frequency sound waves to produce pictures of the interior of the body. It may aid in confirming the existence of a hernia, determining its size and location, and detecting consequences such as intestinal blockage.

MRI and CT scans give more comprehensive pictures of the hernia and adjacent tissues, enabling doctors to determine the extent of the hernia and design the surgical approach appropriately. These imaging studies may be especially effective for complicated or recurring hernias.

Preparing Mentally And Physically For Surgery

Preparing emotionally and physically for hernia repair surgery is critical for a positive result and a seamless recovery. Mental preparation is comprehending the surgical process, its risks and problems, and setting reasonable expectations for the result.

It is natural to feel scared or apprehensive before surgery, but speaking with your healthcare professional, asking questions, and getting support from friends and family may help reduce some of these fears.

Physical preparation for surgery may include lifestyle changes such as stopping smoking, eating a nutritious diet, and remaining active to improve your general health and body's capacity to recover following surgery.

Additionally, your healthcare professional may give you particular advice to follow in the days coming up to surgery, such as fasting before the operation and avoiding certain drugs that might raise the risk of bleeding.

By actively participating in your preoperative preparation, you may help assure the best possible result and a speedier recovery process after hernia repair surgery.

CHAPTER 4

Inguinal Hernia Repair

Anatomy Of The Inguinal Region

Understanding the anatomy of the inguinal area is critical to understanding inguinal hernias and their correction. The inguinal area is found in the lower abdomen, right above the groin. It contains a variety of components such as muscles, blood vessels, nerves, and the inguinal canal. The inguinal canal is a tube that permits tissues such as the spermatic cord in males and the round ligament in women to go from the belly to the genitalia.

Hernias may form in this intricate network of tissues when the abdominal wall muscles weaken or rupture, enabling abdominal contents like fat or intestines to protrude through. Inguinal hernias develop in the inguinal canal or around the inguinal ring, which is a hole in the abdominal wall.

Common Causes Of Inguinal Hernias

Inguinal hernias may occur for a variety of reasons, but the most frequent cause is increased pressure in the abdomen. This pressure may be caused by lifting heavy things, straining during bowel motions or urination, prolonged coughing, obesity, pregnancy, or even a hereditary predisposition to weak stomach walls.

Other contributing causes may include past abdominal operations, muscular weakness from age, and disorders that raise intra-abdominal pressure, such as persistent constipation.

Surgical Procedures For Inguinal Hernia Repair

Inguinal hernia repair is performed using a variety of surgical procedures, each with its own set of pros and disadvantages. There are two basic approaches: open surgery and laparoscopic (minimally invasive) surgery.

Open surgery involves the surgeon making an incision directly over the hernia location. The projecting tissue is pulled back into place, and the weakening abdominal wall is reinforced with sutures or synthetic mesh. This approach provides for direct sight of the hernia and surrounding tissues, making it ideal for complicated hernias or situations where laparoscopic surgery is not an option.

Laparoscopic surgery includes making many tiny incisions in the belly to insert a camera (laparoscope) and specialized surgical equipment. The surgeon next fixes the hernia using mesh, guided by views from the camera on a monitor. Laparoscopic surgery has advantages over open surgery, including smaller incisions, less postoperative discomfort, and shorter recovery periods.

Recovery And Aftercare After Inguinal Hernia Repair

Recovery and postoperative care are critical components of inguinal hernia surgery to guarantee proper healing and avoid problems. Following surgery, patients are often observed in a recovery area until they are stable enough to return home. Pain treatment, rest, and adequate wound care instructions are offered to alleviate pain and lower the risk of infection.

Patients are advised to avoid intense activity, heavy lifting, and driving for the duration suggested by their surgeon. A gradual return to regular activities is urged, with particular guidance for resuming exercise and job tasks.

Follow-up sessions are planned to monitor the healing process and treat any issues or difficulties that may emerge. To get the greatest results after inguinal hernia repair surgery, patients must follow their postoperative care recommendations and attend all follow-up sessions.

CHAPTER 5

Umbilical And Ventral Hernia Repair

Understanding Umbilical And Ventral Hernias

Umbilical and ventral hernias are typical disorders in which abdominal tissue protrudes via weak points in the abdominal wall. Understanding the anatomy of these hernias is critical for comprehending the healing procedure.

Anatomy of umbilical and ventral hernias

Umbilical hernias are characterized by the protrusion of abdominal tissue through the umbilical ring, which is often caused by inadequate closure of the umbilical hole after delivery. Ventral hernias, on the other hand, may arise anywhere along the anterior abdominal wall and are often caused by weak abdominal muscles.

Surgical Treatments For Umbilical And Ventral Hernias

Several surgical procedures are available for correcting umbilical and ventral hernias, each suited to the patient's specific condition and hernia severity.

Laparoscopic Repair

Laparoscopic repair entails creating tiny abdominal incisions through which a laparoscope and specialized surgical equipment are placed. This less invasive procedure provides for a faster recovery and less postoperative discomfort than standard open surgery.

Open Repair.

Open repair, also known as tension-free mesh repair, is another popular method for healing umbilical and ventral hernia. This technique involves making a bigger incision right over the hernia and inserting a synthetic mesh to rebuild the fragile abdominal wall.

This method has great long-term outcomes and is especially successful on bigger hernias.

Complications Of These Types Of Hernias

While hernia repair surgery is typically safe, there are certain risks linked with both the ailment and the surgical process.

Complications from untreated hernias

Untreated umbilical and ventral hernias may cause a variety of consequences, including intestinal obstruction, strangling of the herniated tissue, and incarceration, in which the hernia gets stuck and cannot be moved back into place.

Surgical complications

Infection, bleeding, and mesh-related concerns including migration or erosion are all potential complications of hernia repair surgery.

However, with adequate surgical technique and postoperative care, these issues may often be avoided.

Rehabilitation And Recovery Following Surgery

Rehabilitation and rehabilitation after umbilical and ventral hernia surgery are critical for improving outcomes and avoiding recurrence.

Post-operative Care

After surgery, patients should gradually resume regular activities while avoiding heavy lifting and intense activity for many weeks. Pain management and wound care are particularly important during the first healing phase.

Long-term follow-up

Regular follow-up meetings with the surgeon are advised to check recovery and identify any symptoms of recurrence or problems.

Furthermore, living a healthy lifestyle, such as keeping a healthy weight and avoiding activities that strain the abdominal muscles, may help prevent future hernias.

Understanding the differences between umbilical and ventral hernias, the surgical choices for treatment, possible consequences, and the need for rehabilitation and long-term follow-up is critical to properly treating these frequent abdominal disorders.

CHAPTER 6

Femoral Hernia Repair

Overview Of Femoral Hernias

Femoral hernias are hernias that develop in the groin region. Femoral hernias are different from inguinal hernias in that they protrude via the femoral canal, which is a channel near the groin. These hernias are more frequent in women, particularly those who have been pregnant or given birth.

Obesity, hard lifting, straining during bowel motions, or even standing for an extended length of time may all cause femoral hernias. They often appear as a bulge or lump in the groin region, which may be uncomfortable or unpleasant to touch. If left untreated, femoral hernias may cause major consequences such as intestinal blockage or strangulation, in which blood supply to the herniated tissue is interrupted.

Surgical Approach To Repairing Femoral Hernia

A femoral hernia is often repaired surgically. The surgical technique may differ based on the hernia's size and severity, as well as the patient's general condition.

Herniorrhaphy is a commonly used surgical method for treating femoral hernias. This technique involves the physician making an incision near the hernia and pushing the bulging tissue back into place. They next fix the compromised region with sutures or a mesh patch to prevent the hernia from reoccurring.

Another option is laparoscopic hernia repair, which involves making numerous small incisions and repairing the hernia from inside the belly using a tiny camera and specialized surgical equipment.

Compared to conventional open surgery, this minimally invasive procedure usually results in less postoperative discomfort and a quicker recovery period.

Risks And Complications For Femoral Hernias

While femoral hernia repair is typically safe, surgery does include certain risks and problems. Infection, hemorrhage, nerve injury, and hernia recurrence are all possible complications.

In comparison to other forms of hernias, femoral hernias are more likely to result in imprisonment and strangulation. Incarceration occurs when the herniated tissue gets caught in the femoral canal, while strangulation occurs when the blood supply to the hernia is disrupted. Both of these issues need prompt medical treatment and, in some cases, emergent surgery to avoid catastrophic consequences.

Rehabilitation And Postoperative Care For Femoral Hernia Repair

Recovery following femoral hernia repair surgery often entails rest and restricted physical activity. Patients may suffer soreness, edema, or bruising in the groin region, which may be treated with pain relievers and cold packs.

Patients must follow their surgeon's postoperative care recommendations, which may include avoiding heavy lifting, vigorous activities, or driving for a certain length of time. Patients may gradually resume regular activities as they recuperate, but they must listen to their bodies and avoid overexertion too soon.

Physical therapy or light exercises may also be prescribed to strengthen the abdominal muscles and aid in overall rehabilitation. Patients should attend all follow-up sessions with their surgeon to keep track of their progress and address any concerns or difficulties that may emerge throughout the healing period.

CHAPTER 7

Laparoscopic Hernia Repair Techniques

Introduction To Laparoscopic Surgery

Laparoscopic surgery, often known as minimally invasive surgery, has transformed the medical industry by providing less invasive alternatives to standard open procedures. Instead of massive incisions, laparoscopic surgeries use tiny incisions to introduce specialized devices and a camera. This equipment enables surgeons to conduct difficult treatments with more accuracy while watching a magnified, high-resolution picture of the surgical site on a display.

One of the most important components of laparoscopic surgery is the use of a laparoscope, which is a thin, flexible tube with a camera and light source. This equipment acts as the surgeon's eyes within the body, allowing a good view of interior organs and tissues. Furthermore, specialized equipment such as graspers, scissors, and dissectors are utilized to manipulate tissues and execute surgical procedures with little harm to adjacent structures.

Advantages Of Laparoscopic Hernia Repair

Laparoscopic hernia surgery has various benefits over conventional open hernia repair methods. For starters, since it includes fewer incisions, patients usually have less postoperative discomfort and scarring, resulting in a faster recovery period. This may lead to shorter hospital stays and a speedier return to routine activities like work and exercise.

Furthermore, the minimally invasive nature of laparoscopic hernia treatment lowers the risk of consequences such as wound infections and hernia recurrence. Avoiding big incisions and limiting impact on surrounding tissues reduces the risk of nerve damage and persistent pain after surgery. Furthermore, the greater visibility given by the laparoscope enables more accurate mesh insertion to repair the fragile abdominal wall, lowering the risk of future hernias.

Another benefit of laparoscopic hernia treatment is better cosmetic results. Smaller incisions result in fewer visible scars, which may be especially advantageous for patients worried about the cosmetic effect of surgery. Overall, these benefits make laparoscopic hernia repair an appealing alternative for patients who want a quicker, less painful recovery with a lower risk of complications.

Techniques And Instruments For Laparoscopic Hernia Repair

Several procedures may be employed in laparoscopic hernia repair, including transabdominal preperitoneal (TAPP) and completely extraperitoneal (TEP) approaches. Both methods involve the surgeon making tiny incisions around the hernia site and inserting the laparoscope and specialized equipment into the abdominal cavity.

During a TAPP repair, the peritoneum (the thin membrane that lines the abdominal cavity) is cut, providing access to the herniated sac. The sac is subsequently decreased, and a mesh patch is applied to the hernia defect to strengthen the abdominal wall. The peritoneum is subsequently closed over the mesh, and the wounds are sealed with sutures or surgical glue.

A TEP repair does not involve entering the peritoneum, and the mesh is put beneath the peritoneum and abdominal muscles. This approach avoids the possible difficulties of accessing the peritoneal cavity and may be favored in certain cases, such as bilateral hernias or individuals with a history of intra-abdominal surgery.

Various specialized equipment are utilized during laparoscopic hernia surgery to help in dissection, mesh implantation, and wound closure. This equipment may include graspers, scissors, dissectors, and staplers, all of which are intended to accomplish specialized jobs precisely and efficiently. Furthermore, modern technology such as robotic-assisted surgery may be employed to improve the surgeon's skills and patient outcomes.

Recovery And Results Of Laparoscopic Hernia Repair

When compared to conventional open surgery, laparoscopic hernia treatment often results in a quicker and less painful recovery. Patients may have moderate discomfort and soreness at the incision sites, which may typically be treated with over-the-counter pain relievers. Most patients may resume their usual activities within a few days to a week after surgery, although vigorous activity and heavy lifting should be avoided for several weeks to allow for adequate recovery.

Laparoscopic hernia repair has been demonstrated to provide equivalent or even better results than open surgery. Laparoscopic procedures have been shown in studies to reduce the risk of postoperative complications such as wound infections and hernia recurrence. Furthermore, patients often express greater satisfaction with the cosmetic outcomes of laparoscopic surgery owing to fewer incisions and less visible scars.

Overall, laparoscopic hernia treatment has many benefits over conventional open procedures, such as speedier recovery, less discomfort, and better esthetic results. Using modern laparoscopic procedures and tools, surgeons may successfully treat hernias with minimum stress to surrounding tissues, resulting in greater patient results and satisfaction.

CHAPTER 8

Open Hernia Repair Techniques

Traditional Open Hernia Repair Methods

Traditional open hernia repair procedures have been used for decades to treat hernias, providing patients with solid remedies. One frequent procedure is tension-free repair, which involves removing the hernia sac and reinforcing the defect with mesh. Another option is to heal the hernia with sutures alone, without employing mesh. Each technique has its own set of indications, and the decision is based on considerations such as the size and location of the hernia, the patient's medical history, and the surgeon's preference.

Tension-free repair involves the surgeon making an incision around the hernia site and delicately dissecting the tissue to reveal the hernia sac. The sac is then removed, and any protruding tissue is put back into position. A synthetic mesh is subsequently put over the defect and held in place with sutures or surgical staples. This approach distributes strain across the healing site, lowering the likelihood of recurrence.

Suture repair, on the other hand, uses sutures to close the hernia defect directly. This procedure is most often utilized for minor hernias or when mesh installation is not an option. While it is easier than tension-free repair, it has a greater chance of recurrence, particularly for bigger hernias or those located in high-tension locations such as the inguinal region.

The Pros And Disadvantages Of Open Hernia Repair

Open hernia repair has various benefits over other procedures, making it a better option in some instances. One significant benefit is the ability to see directly into the hernia sac and surrounding tissue, allowing for a comprehensive assessment and exact treatment.

This may lead to decreased recurrence rates compared to laparoscopic procedures, particularly for complicated hernias.

Furthermore, open repair provides simpler access to the hernia site, making it appropriate for individuals with extensive scar tissue or past abdominal procedures. It also gives tactile input to the surgeon, allowing for more precise mesh or suture insertion. Furthermore, open repair is frequently less expensive than laparoscopic procedures, making it available to a broader spectrum of patients.

However, open hernia repair has several downsides. The treatment often needs a wider incision than laparoscopic surgery, which results in more postoperative discomfort and lengthier recovery durations. Patients may feel pain at the incision site and have restricted movement during the early healing phase. Furthermore, there is a tiny chance of wound problems like infection or hernia recurrence, although these are uncommon with adequate surgical technique and postoperative care.

Surgical Procedure For Open Hernia Repair

The surgical method for open hernia repair starts with the patient being comfortably positioned on the operating table and given an anesthetic. The surgeon next makes an incision around the hernia location, being cautious to avoid any major blood vessels or nerves. Once revealed, the hernia sac is carefully dissected and either removed or reinserted into the abdominal cavity.

Depending on the healing procedure used, the surgeon will next strengthen the defect using mesh or sutures. For tension-free repair, a synthetic mesh is cut to suit the defect and put over the weak spot. The mesh is subsequently fixed in place with absorbable sutures or surgical staples.

When sutures are used alone, the defect is carefully repaired with strong, non-absorbable stitches.

After the repair is done, the incision is closed with sutures or surgical staples, and a sterile dressing is put on the wound. After being observed in the recovery room, the patient is released home with postoperative care instructions.

Postoperative Care And Recovery Following Open Hernia Repair

Postoperative care is critical for a successful recovery after open hernia surgery. Patients should relax and avoid heavy activity for the first several days after surgery to enable the incision site to heal properly. They may feel soreness, bruising, and swelling around the surgery site, which may be treated with over-the-counter pain relievers and cold packs.

Patients should follow their surgeon's wound care guidelines, which include keeping the incision clean and dry and avoiding activities that impose tension on the abdominal muscles. They should also look for indications of infection, such as increased redness, swelling, or drainage from the incision site, and tell their doctor if any concerns occur.

Patients may gradually resume modest activities and raise the amount of physical effort as tolerated. However, hard lifting and vigorous activity should be avoided for many weeks to minimize problems and encourage normal recovery. Most patients may resume regular daily activities within a few weeks, although complete recovery may take many months.

Follow-up consultations with the surgeon have been set to evaluate the healing process and handle any concerns or issues that may emerge. Patients who follow postoperative care recommendations and attend follow-up consultations should anticipate a positive result and long-term relief from hernia symptoms.

CHAPTER 9

Complications And Risks

Possible Complications Of Hernia Repair Surgery

When having hernia repair surgery, it is important to be informed of any possible problems that may occur during or after the treatment. While these consequences are uncommon, recognizing them may help you make better choices and plan for your recovery.

Infection

Infection is a possible consequence of hernia repair surgery. While surgeons make efforts to reduce the risk of infection, it may nevertheless occur in certain circumstances.

Infections may cause redness, swelling, fever, or drainage at the surgical site. In extreme instances, fever and chills may accompany the illness.

To reduce the risk of infection, surgeons usually provide antibiotics before and after surgery. Additionally, adhering to good wound care and cleanliness standards might help avoid infections. To limit the risk of problems, strictly adhere to your surgeon's post-operative recommendations.

Recurrence Of Hernia

Despite successful hernia repair surgery, there is a risk of recurrence. Recurrence may occur for a variety of reasons, including poor tissue recovery, undue strain on the surgery site, or the formation of a new hernia in the same area. While recurrence rates vary based on the kind of hernia and surgical procedure utilized, it is critical to watch for indicators of recurrence, such as bulging or pain at the prior hernia site.

To lessen the chance of hernia recurrence, surgeons may use mesh to strengthen the treated tissue or use minimally invasive procedures that result in fewer problems. However, even with these precautions, recurrence may occur in certain situations. Regular follow-up sessions with your surgeon will help you track your recovery and spot any symptoms of recurrence early.

Chronic Pain And Other Long-Term Risks

Chronic discomfort is another possible hazard of hernia repair surgery, albeit less frequent than infection or recurrence. Some patients may endure ongoing pain or sensitivity at the surgery site, affecting their quality of life. Chronic discomfort following hernia repair surgery might be caused by nerve injury, scar tissue development, or mesh-related complications.

To treat persistent pain, surgeons may offer pain management techniques such as medication, physical therapy, or nerve blocks. In certain circumstances, further surgical procedures may be required to relieve chronic discomfort.

Aside from persistent discomfort, hernia repair surgery has additional long-term hazards. These may include anesthesia-related complications such as allergic reactions or breathing difficulties, as well as possible organ or tissue damage during the surgical process.

While problems are possible with any surgical operation, hernia repair surgery is usually regarded as safe and beneficial for the majority of patients. Understanding the possible risks and adopting proactive actions to reduce risk can allow you to undertake hernia repair surgery with confidence and achieve a positive result.

CHAPTER 10

Post-Operative Care And Recovery

Immediate Postoperative Care At The Hospital

Immediate postoperative care after hernia repair surgery is critical for a successful recovery. After waking up from anesthesia, patients are often carefully followed in the recovery room by qualified medical personnel. Vital indicators such as heart rate, blood pressure, and oxygen saturation are monitored to maintain stability. Pain treatment starts immediately, with drugs given as required to keep the patient comfortable.

Once the patient has stabilized, they may be moved to a hospital room for additional observation. During this phase, the medical team will keep an eye out for any symptoms of problems such as bleeding, infection, or anesthesia-related bad effects. Patients are recommended to relax and adhere to any special advice issued by their surgeon or medical team.

If patients are unable to accept oral intake during the initial postoperative period, they may be given intravenous fluids to keep them hydrated and fed. As the patient's health improves, they may move to a clear liquid diet, followed by solid meals as tolerated.

Nurses and other healthcare workers play an important role in teaching patients about their healing process at this time. They provide advice on wound care, activity limits, and symptoms of possible issues to look out for after you leave the oshpital.

Pain Management Strategies

Pain management is an essential part of postoperative therapy after hernia repair surgery. Several treatments are used to assist patients in managing pain and enhance healing throughout the recovery phase.

Patients are often given pain medicines right after surgery, such as acetaminophen, nonsteroidal anti-inflammatory drugs (NSAIDs), or opioids for more severe pain. These drugs may be given orally, intravenously, or via other means, depending on the patient's requirements and the surgeon's recommendations.

In addition to pharmaceutical therapies, non-drug pain management strategies may be used. These may include applying cold packs to the surgery site to minimize swelling and numbness, using compression garments or abdominal binders for support, and practicing relaxation methods such as deep breathing exercises or guided imagery.

Patients should talk honestly with their healthcare providers about their pain levels and any concerns they have about pain treatment. Individual demands and preferences may need dose adjustments or the use of alternative therapy.

Physical Activity And Return To Normal Routine

Physical exercise is important in the recovery process after hernia repair surgery, but a mix of rest and movement is required to avoid problems and improve healing. While patients should avoid vigorous activity and heavy lifting in the initial postoperative period, moderate movement and mild exercise may help with circulation and recuperation.

Patients are often urged to take brief walks about the home or hospital ward to help avoid blood clots and improve bowel function. As their rehabilitation develops, individuals may progressively increase the time and intensity of their physical activities with the help of their medical team.

Returning to typical everyday activities such as work, driving, and housework will depend on the kind of hernia repair done, the individual's healing process, and any special instructions supplied by the surgeon.

Most patients should anticipate to resume modest activities within a few days to a week after surgery, with complete recovery requiring several weeks or months.

Patients must listen to their bodies and avoid pushing themselves too hard throughout the rehabilitation process. Overexertion might raise the risk of problems and lengthen the healing process. Before resuming any vigorous activities, consult with your surgeon or healthcare practitioner to ensure a safe and effective recovery.

Long-Term Follow-Up And Monitoring

Long-term follow-up and monitoring are critical components of hernia repair surgery because they allow you to evaluate the procedure's progress, watch for any complications, and treat any remaining concerns or difficulties.

Patients usually have follow-up visits with their surgeon or healthcare provider in the weeks and months after surgery. During these appointments, the surgical incision site will be examined for healing progress, and the patient's concerns or queries will be addressed.

In addition to in-person checkups, patients may undergo imaging tests such as ultrasounds or CT scans to assess the integrity of the surgery and identify hernia recurrence. Patients must attend all planned follow-up visits and quickly report any changes or symptoms to their healthcare provider.

Beyond the initial healing phase, patients are recommended to live a healthy lifestyle that includes regular exercise, a balanced diet, and avoiding smoking or excessive alcohol use to improve general health and limit the chance of hernia recurrence or complications. Patients who follow these long-term instructions and remain proactive in their treatment may improve their results and recover well after hernia repair surgery.

Conclusion

Finally, both patients and healthcare providers benefit from a thorough grasp of hernia repair. Throughout this book, we've covered the complexity of hernias, including their causes, symptoms, and treatment choices. We've looked at the necessity of early detection and individualized treatment options based on unique patient characteristics.

Recognizing the signs and symptoms of a hernia is critical. Understanding these symptoms, which range from the typical bulge to discomfort or pain, might lead people to seek medical assistance as soon as possible, perhaps averting difficulties later.

Second, knowing the many forms of hernias is critical. Whether inguinal, femoral, umbilical, or incisional, each variety poses unique obstacles and necessitates distinct healing methods.

Third, we investigated the various treatment options for hernias, which ranged from careful waiting and lifestyle changes to surgical intervention. Some hernias may be treated conservatively, while others need surgical correction to avoid potentially serious consequences including intestinal blockage or strangling.

We've also examined the progression of hernia repair treatments, from conventional open surgery to less invasive approaches like laparoscopic and robotic-assisted operations. These developments have resulted in dramatically decreased postoperative pain, shorter recovery periods, and better overall patient outcomes.

In addition, we've emphasized the need for patient education and collaborative decision-making in hernia care. Empowering patients with information about their disease and including them in treatment choices increases a feeling of control over their health and improves adherence to treatment programs.

Furthermore, we've stressed the need for a multidisciplinary approach to hernia treatment, with surgeons, primary care doctors, nurses, and other healthcare professionals working together to provide complete, patient-centered care.

Finally, although hernias may be serious health problems, advances in detection and treatment have significantly improved results for those who suffer from them. Understanding the complexities of hernia repair allows patients to make more educated choices regarding their treatment, resulting in improved overall health and well-being. Continued research and innovation in this sector will surely increase our capacity to successfully treat hernias and improve patients' quality of life throughout the globe.

THE END

Made in the USA
Las Vegas, NV
10 September 2024